YOUR KNOWLEDGE HAS VALUE

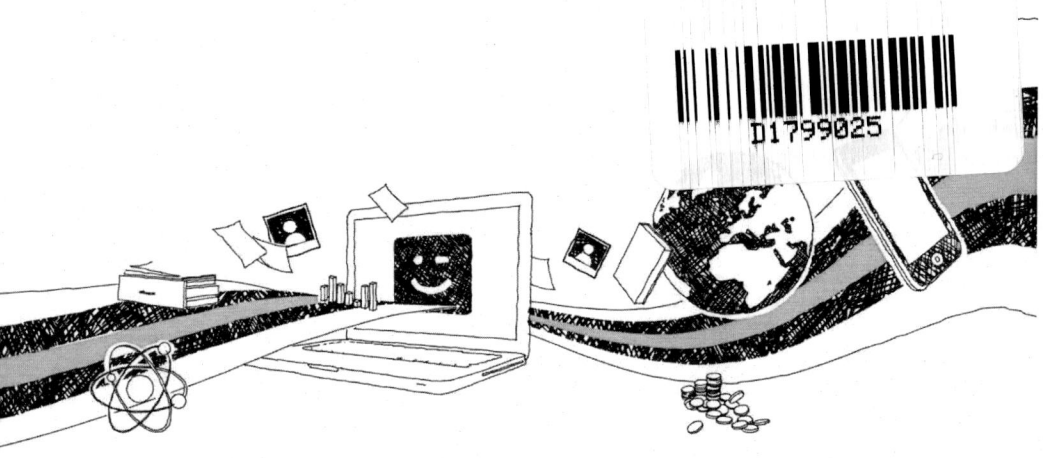

- We will publish your bachelor's and master's thesis, essays and papers

- Your own eBook and book - sold worldwide in all relevant shops

- Earn money with each sale

Upload your text at www.GRIN.com
and publish for free

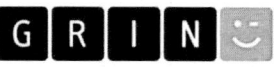

Miriam Mennen

International Trade and Finance - Pharmaceutical Industry in Germany

Research and Development - Innovation and Knowledge Creation

GRIN Verlag

Bibliografische Information der Deutschen Nationalbibliothek:

Die Deutsche Bibliothek verzeichnet diese Publikation in der Deutschen National-
bibliografie; detaillierte bibliografische Daten sind im Internet über http://dnb.d-
nb.de/ abrufbar.

Dieses Werk sowie alle darin enthaltenen einzelnen Beiträge und Abbildungen
sind urheberrechtlich geschützt. Jede Verwertung, die nicht ausdrücklich vom
Urheberrechtsschutz zugelassen ist, bedarf der vorherigen Zustimmung des Verla-
ges. Das gilt insbesondere für Vervielfältigungen, Bearbeitungen, Übersetzungen,
Mikroverfilmungen, Auswertungen durch Datenbanken und für die Einspeicherung
und Verarbeitung in elektronische Systeme. Alle Rechte, auch die des auszugsweisen
Nachdrucks, der fotomechanischen Wiedergabe (einschließlich Mikrokopie) sowie
der Auswertung durch Datenbanken oder ähnliche Einrichtungen, vorbehalten.

Imprint:

Copyright © 2006 GRIN Verlag GmbH
Druck und Bindung: Books on Demand GmbH, Norderstedt Germany
ISBN: 978-3-640-56853-6

This book at GRIN:

http://www.grin.com/en/e-book/145357/international-trade-and-finance-pharma-
ceutical-industry-in-germany

MA International Management

Full Time Degree

Assignment

International Trade and Finance

APCM09

Name: Miriam Mennen

Submission date: 10th June 2006

Table of Contents

1. Introduction

According to Krugman (1992, p.17), *"there was never a time when the study of international economics was as important as it is today"*. Through international trade in goods and services and the international flows of money, the extent of markets is widened in order to offer the consumer a larger variety of products. Along with Bolisani and Scarso (1996), *"global competition urges firms not only to develop a strong commercial presence in the world market, but also to assume an international configuration with regard to operations."*

Van Marrewijk (2002) argues that it increases the *"welfare of a nation through the love-of-variety effect for final goods or raises production through increased specialization leading to positive production externalities"*. This, of course, raises the competition of different companies in different nations towards quality improvements and innovation which results in increasing efforts in Research and Development (R&D). Grossman and Helpman (1991) demonstrated in their approach that it is more complex to improve quality than increase product variety, even though they have similar profitable results. Nevertheless, it can be assumed that by innovation through more engagement in R&D the operating profit will be increased.

The WTO is one of today's organisation dealing with international trade issues and basically assuring and emphasising free global trade, but during its formation also other regional trade agreements between countries occurred (regionalism). Soon the fear of a swift from multilateralism towards regionalism and protectionism appeared which was constituted by Krugman's framework of intra-industry trade, which takes place *"in order to take advantage of important economies of scale in production"*. Therefore, intra-industry trade became of particular importance with the removal of tariffs and trade barriers. (Salvatore, 2004, p.171)

However, it can be said that trade between nations *"is a form of exchange which contributes to increased wealth, rising living standards and the sustained economic development of trading nations"*. (Lawler and Seddighi, 2001)

This paper will firstly analyse the importance of R&D, its global dimension and its future trends. Furthermore, the emphasis by nations put on investment in knowledge will be explained. The second part then outlines the main economic theories concerning innovation and knowledge creation. Finally, Germany and its pharmaceutical industry will be taken as an example to illustrate the dimensions of investment in R&D and its outcomes.

2. Research and Development & Knowledge Creation

According to the United Nations (2006), Research and Development can be defined as "*any creative systematic activity undertaken in order to increase the stock of knowledge, including knowledge of man, culture and society, and the use of this knowledge to devise new applications.*" This also includes the research applied in such fields as "*agriculture, medicine, industrial chemistry, and experimental development work leading to new devices, products or processes.*"

Today's business environment indicates a high level of integration with rapid technological change which creates a new situation for competing companies. According to 'World-wide R&D' (2006), the global business climate has continued to improve in overall sales growth, profitability and R&D levels, measured among the 1,000 largest companies by R&D investment. Tubbs (2005) argues that R&D becomes more and more important for generating new products providing a competitive advantage because when a firm invests relatively less in R&D compared to its competitors, it will soon lose the competitive edge and has to increase lower value added products. Therefore, a company's competitiveness is highly reliant on its "*capacity to innovate and create new value*". (Kastelli, 2006) Knowledge creation, in this context, can be defined as the capability of a firm, to create new knowledge, circulate it throughout company and exemplify it in its product, services and systems (Nonaka and Takeushi, 1995).

Besides using their own knowledge competencies, firms also network with their environment in order to increase skills with complementary competencies of others. (Kastelli, 2006)

Figure1 illustrates the necessity of R&D investment for R&D-intensive companies and the size of these investments for the three largest R&D intensive sectors.

Sector	R&D as % Sales	Capex as % of Sales	Cost of Funds as % of Sales (sum of interest and dividends)	Operating Profit as % Sales
Pharmaceuticals	15	5.2	7	19.5
IT - Hardware	8.6	5.2	1.8	8
Software	10.7	3.6	2	18.5

Figure1. R&D compared to key company expenses for 3 R&D-intensive sectors
Source: Tubbs, 2005

Global R&D

Over the past decade, the expenditure on R&D has been rising constantly to US $ 829.9 billion in 2002 which indicates that 1.7 % of the worlds GDP is spend on R&D. (Unesco Science Report, 2005)

The OECD Factbook (2006) states, that the "*expenditure on Research and Development (R&D) is a key indicator of government and private sector efforts to obtain competitive advantage in science and technology.*" The gross domestic expenditure on research and development, also referred to as GERD, then indicates the "*total expenditure on R&D performed on the national territory*" It is used for an international comparison and includes all local firms and laboratories and excludes financial expenditure which is invested abroad. (Federal Ministry of Education and Research, 2005)

Gross domestic expenditure on R&D
As a percentage (2004, latest available year)

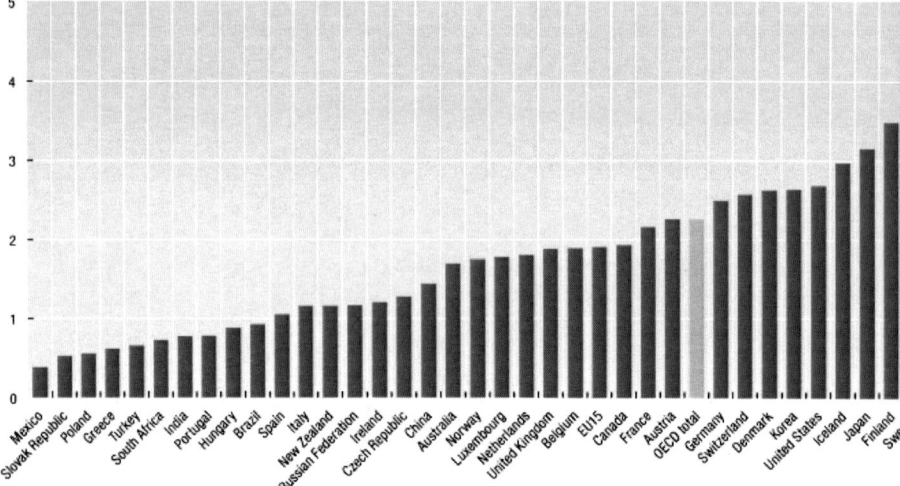

Figure 2. Gross Domestic Expenditure on R&D
Source: OECD Factbook, 2006

It can be seen in Figure 2, that R&D in 2003 summed up to 2.3 % of GDP of the total OECD countries. According to the OECD Factbook (2006), it should be taken into consideration that several countries like Japan, the Netherlands, Norway and the US have advanced their R&D activities in the service sector or in a higher education.

R&D trends
It can be argued that gross domestic expenditure on R&D increased in Japan (from 2.96 % in 2000 to 3.15 % in 2003) and, even though a little lesser, in the European Union (from 1.87 % to 1.91 % in 2003), whereas it decreased in the United States (from 2.74% in 2000 to 2.68 % in 2004). With Iceland (2.97 % in 2003) bordering the 3 % mark, Japan (3.15 %), Finland (3.48 %) and Sweden (3.98 %) are the only OECD countries in which the R&D intensity surpassed the 3 % mark in 2003. Compared over the period from 1981 till 2003, Portugal (0.30 % to 0.78 %), Iceland (0.64 % to 2.97 %) and Turkey (0.32 % in 1990 to 0.66 % in 2003) have been growing the fastest in terms of their R&D expenditure. (OECD Factbook, 2006, see Appendix 1)

With US $ 307.2 billion, North America has spent 37.0 % in 2002 of the world gross expenditure on R&D and is therefore the main investor in knowledge creation, even though it has a little decreased since 1990 (38.2 %).
(UIS Bulletin on Science and Technology Statistics, 2004)

As stated in Figure 3, it is crucial to see that Asia, with 31.5 %, took over Europe (27.3 %) in its world shares of GERD. According to the above stated facts, the US gross domestic expenditure on R&D was decreasing between 2000 and 2004, whereas Japans GERD was increasing tremendously by almost 0.2 % within the last 4 years. This then links us to the question whether the US, Japan and some northern European countries can keep their dominance in knowledge creation or if the wealth gained from R&D activities will be shared among a larger number of countries and "a more balanced situation is emerging". (Unesco Science Report, 2005)

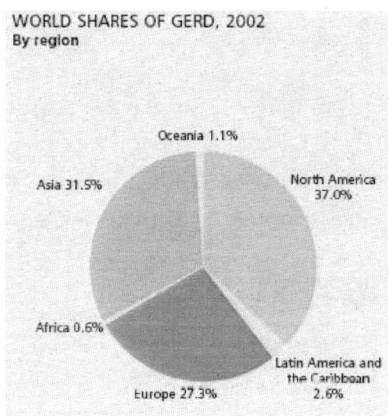

Figure 3. World Shares of GERD in 2002
Source: Unesco Science Report, 2005

Investment in Knowledge

"Investment in knowledge is defined and calculated as the sum of expenditure on R&D, on total higher education (public and private) and on software." (OECD Factbook, 2006)

Investment in knowledge
As a percentage of GDP (2002, latest available year)

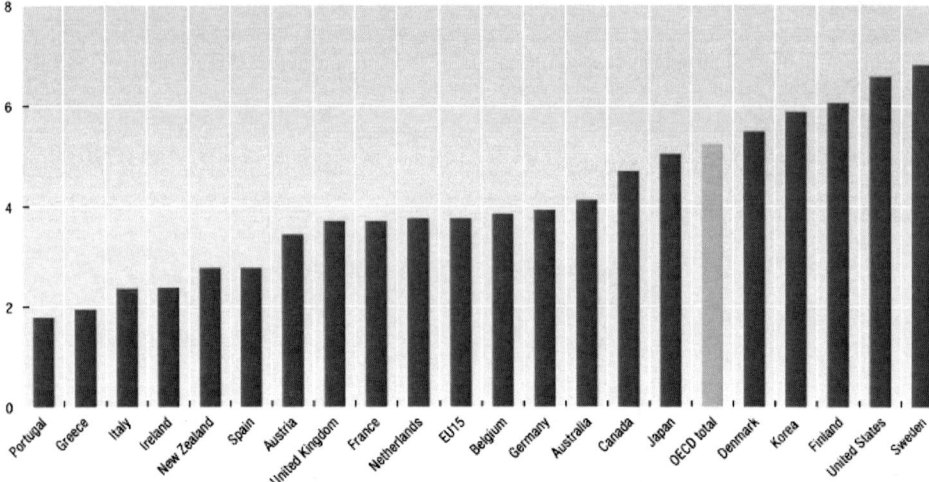

Figure 4. Investment in Knowledge in 2002
Source: OECD Factbook, 2006

As shown in Figure 4, Sweden has with 6.8 % the highest investment in knowledge. Nevertheless, the US (5.4 % in 1994 to 6.6 % in 2002) as well as Japan (3.9 % in 1994 to 5.0 % in 2002) performed a higher increase towards a knowledge-based economy than most of the European nations (EU15 = 3.8 %). According to the OECD Factbook (2006), it can be argued that the most common reason for an increased investment in knowledge, over the past decade, was the rising expenditure on software.

However, the OECD Factbook (2006) identified that the industries with the highest insensitivity of R&D are information technology (soft & hardware) (USA), aerospace (UK), electronics (Japan), telecommunication (Finland) and pharmaceuticals (UK, Germany, USA).

Looking at the future, it can be analysed that globally countries are investing into building innovation capacity in order to push economic growth. Europe in general has a declining level of R&D investment, but it will still remain strong in their key sectors. Latin America on the other side will intensify its investment in the pharmaceutical and chemical sectors. Furthermore Asia and especially Korea will increase their R&D expenditure enormously, focusing on telecommunications, electronics and computers. (Ambrecht, 2006)

Figure 5 outlines some selected countries in order to demonstrate the difference between European key players; Germany, France and the UK, which invested less than 4 % and the high investing countries in knowledge; Finland, Sweden and the US, which spend more than 6 % of GDP in 2002.

Investment in knowledge for selected countries
As a percentage of GDP

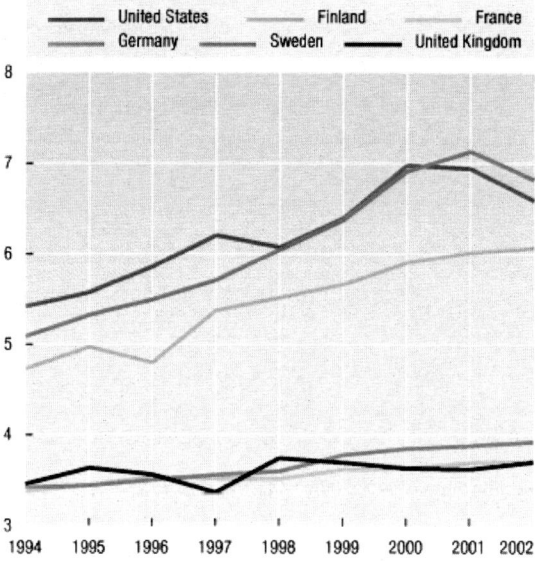

Figure 5. Development of Investment in Knowledge for selected countries
Source: OECD Factbook, 2006

Concluding, it can be said that most developing countries failed in involving themselves in global knowledge creation systems which puts them at the best in the position of a knowledge developing country in terms of competitiveness. It is crucial to realise that, the more advanced the technology and its capabilities are, the more countries are able to sustain competitive while shifting knowledge development to lower skilled countries. Instead of obtaining technology from developed countries, developing countries have to learn to innovate in order to be part of the knowledge creation process. (World Investment Report 2005)

3. Economic Theories

Nowadays, the phenomenon of intra-industry trade is dominating world trade, which can be defined as the simultaneously trade between countries within the same industry. This topic was of particular relevance for several theoretical economists, like Pieter Verdoorn (1960), Bela Balassa (1966) or Peter Lloyd (1975), because all theories of comparative advantage developed till then could not explain intra-industry trade. (van Marrewijk, 2002) It can be said that comparative advantage theories, like the Heckscher-Ohlin model, focus on differences in endowments like capital, labour or other resources, whereas *"intra-industry trade is based on product differentiation and economies of scale."* As a matter of fact, these theoretical simultaneous goods or services traded by countries are not the same. With intra-industry trade, the demand for similar products is driven by consumers demanding a variety of similar, but not identically goods and services. (Salvatore, 2004)

The H-O theory, which emphasises the differences in the availability of labour, capital and natural resources among nations, the advantages through economies of scale and the dynamics in changes of technology, can be examined by the technological gap and Vernon's (1966) product cycle model. Both models can be seen as an extension to the unchanging H-O model. Whereas the technological gap model, developed by Posner (1961), is based on the introduction of new products through innovation which gives the country or the company a temporary monopoly position, the product cycle gap model by Vernon (1966) gives a further development of this theory. It stresses the need of skilled labour when a new product is introduced and the shift to mass production techniques by less skilled labour when the standardised product gained acceptance. Therefore, comparative advantage moves from the innovating nation, through foreign direct investment, to the less advanced nation with cheaper labour. Vernon furthermore points out, that expensive but labour-saving products are more likely to be introduced to rich nations. Consequently, it is expected from highly industrialised economies to export non-standardised products with *"new and more advanced technologies and import products embodying old or less advanced technologies"*. (Salvatore, 2004, p.179) In 1967, the theory was extended by a new study by Gruber, Mehta and Vernon as they explored a close linkage between the expenditure on R&D and the export performance of a nation. The expenditure on R&D was taken as a substitute for a momentary comparative advantage that states or companies acquire in new manufacturing processes. (Salvatore, 2004, p.180)

According to van Marrewijk (2002), a reason for simultaneously trade is, besides the high level of investment, also the time of innovation and development that it takes for a company to saturate the demand with a domestic production of requirements. Therefore, a theoretical explanation for the phenomenon of intra-industry trade has to include consumer needs, the increasing returns for a company through production of scale of a limited line of products and a competitive market situation. Salvatore (2004) argues that it is crucial for companies in order to lower their unit costs. The nation then imports other desired varieties from other nations. Krugman (1979, 1980) developed a good introduction to international economic action and a theory of growth by determining the extent of intra-industry trade, which can be measure by the Grublel-Lloyd index = 1- (exports-imports) / (exports+imports). An industry indicating an index close to one shows that there is a high level of intra-industry trade as there are almost as many exports as imports. He argues that a bigger market is better able to fulfil customer needs. It can be explained as a sharing of countries' domestic markets, as the consumers obtain products from domestic producers and import from the foreign ones. (van Marrewijk, 2002, p. 183) Due to this demand for diversity in consumption, firms in each of the trading countries have an incentive to import unique varieties from abroad rather than spending another fixed cost and producing those goods locally. (Grossman and Helpman, 1992) However, the main outcome of Krugman's model is that only technological change will lead to capital movement towards the innovating country. Furthermore, knowledge creating countries must continually process their technology in order to *"maintain their real incomes, and not simply just to maintain growth, as argued by Vernon"*. (Lawler and Seddighi, 2001)

Cantwell (1995) however found out that, in contrast to Vernon's original product cycle model, there is an increase towards internationalisation of R&D by knowledge creating countries compared to the 1960s. He suggests that technology leaders should develop *"international intra-firm networks to exploit the locationally differentiated potential of foreign centres of excellence...in order to extend its core technological competence"*. Furthermore, companies should also engage in external inter-firm networks to cooperate and learn from technology-based joint ventures. Therefore, FDI in R&D is constantly increasing through firms' carrying out their R&D abroad which, on the other hand, is leading to concerns about the benefits for the host nations. Even though, the home country is still remaining the most important location for R&D, cross-investments between knowledge centres are also very crucial in terms of innovation. They "*have probably helped to reinforce the existing pattern of geographical specialisation and the importance of these centres as locations for innovation*". Furthermore, Cantwell (1995) is arguing that highly innovating countries create wealth in form of high incomes and demand but technological leadership is also a cause for it.

4.   Germany and the pharmaceutical industry

Germany's pharmaceutical industry will be taken as an example for a knowledge creating country.

Germany has a population of 82.7million and a gross domestic product of US $ 3.00 trillion which indicates a growth rate of 1.6 %, from just 0.8 % in 2005. Whereas Germany's growth rate was declining since the 1990s, it is now recovering its stagnation. With a per capita purchasing power party of
US $ 30.579, it is the largest economy in Europe and the fifth largest in the world after the US, Japan, China and India. Germany, as the worlds biggest export nation (US $ 1.016 trillion) and the second largest import nation (US $ 801 billion) had a trade surplus of US $ 204 billion and can be called a high income country with high living standards. (The Economist, 2006)

Germany is among the world's leading nations in scientific research, innovation and knowledge creation. Its gross domestic expenditure on R&D started increasing steadily, with a growth rate of 21%, from € 40.4 billion in 1995 to € 54.3 billion in 2003, which leads to a percentage of GERD increase from 2.25 % in 1995 to 2.55 % in 2003 (see Appendix 2). According to the objectives of the European Union (Lisbon strategy), around 66 % of the gross domestic expenditure on R&D is financed by industry. (Federal Ministry of Education and Research, 2005)

Additionally, Germany stresses on education and a skilled labour force in order to sustain a knowledge creating country. In Appendix 3 it can be seen that there was an increase in expenditure on education, with a growth rate of 37.5 % from € 7.2 billion (1998) to € 9.9 billion in 2005. (Federal Ministry of Education and Research, 2005) Germany has the capacity to innovate and is promoting it constantly. Therefore, universities and research institutions are encouraged to collaborate directly with the pharmaceutical industry, which is turning out to be very beneficial. (Invest in Germany, 2004)

In the pharmaceutical industry, high expenditures on R&D are necessary to sustain competitive on the global market but also reflect the importance of innovation to the country. The R&D of an innovative pharmaceutical usually takes up to 12 years with an average cost of US $ 800 million. Appendix 4 illustrates that the development of new pharmaceuticals is more costly and labour-intensive than for example the motor-vehicle, the manufacturing or the electric industry in Germany. (VFA, 2006) Therefore, R&D is additionally funded by Germany's federal and state government and the European Union. (Invest in Germany, 2004)

The industry is also characterised by small and medium-sized companies which allow the industry to be more flexible, effective and able to adapt changes in the present market environment. On the other hand, they lack on resources to extend growth which is why cooperation's with foreign firms are formed in order to share resources and strategic skills. (Invest in Germany, 2006)

With the total sales volume of € 23.7 billion and an export rate of 55 %, Germany has a strong pharmaceutical market (see Appendix 5.1) and ranks fourth in per capita sales (see Figure 6) after the US, Japan and France, it still has a decreasing percentage of world sales (see Appendix 5.5). However, the main export partner of Germany is the US and with a steadily growing demand it accounts for 21 % of exports. (Invest in Germany, 2004)

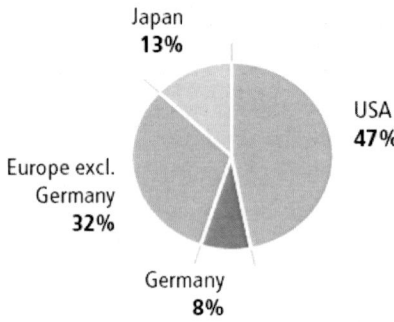

Figure 6: World Sales of Pharmaceuticals
Source: VFA, 2005

Comparing Germany to other European countries, it can be said that there is an extensive increase in R&D investment and pharmaceutical production by countries such as the UK, Denmark and Sweden.

Nevertheless, Germany still remains the most innovative country in Europe as it registers more patents than any other European nation. Additionally, the significance of innovation in the pharmaceutical industry in Germany is mirrored in the R&D expenditure of € 3.82 billion in 2002, which accounts for 15.7 % (see Appendix 4) of their total R&D expenditure (13 % increase from previous year) and the 16,000 people working for pharmaceutical R&D. (Invest in Germany, 2004)

Concerning intra-industry trade, which shows the economic integration between certain economies, it can be said, that for example Germany and Japan have comparable strengths in their bilateral trade. Even though, some IIT index values are quite high (agriculture, intermediate products, cars), the index ranks quite low (0.4) in 2000 in the pharmaceutical industry. (Pascha, 2002)

Concluding, it can be said that Germany is a successful key player in the global pharmaceutical industry concerning innovation and capital spending capacity. The country will continue maintaining a leading rank considering innovation and knowledge creation. Therefore, a set of new reforms, 'Agenda 2010', will be introduced in order to *"remove barriers to investment, cut taxes and social welfare contributions."*

According to the former chancellor, Gerhard Schröder (cited in 'Invest in Germany', 2004), the country is increasing its investment in education, research and technology because *"knowledge based products and services will play an even greater role in determining the economic success of German."*

However, the number of prescriptions for drugs is declining and the inability to compensate this deficit by exports and it becomes questionable if Germans pharmaceutical industry is able to continue its innovation and contribution to the worlds' pharmaceutical progress. (VFA, 2006)

5. Conclusion

By identifying countries like the US or Japan as key players in knowledge creation, it can be assumed that this matches with Krugman's model of intra-industry trade as it includes consumer demands and producers have higher profit margins which results in more resources for knowledge creation (R&D) and investment. Consumers, with their growing demand for innovation, are mostly the reason for economic trends and they also profit from a higher level of knowledge creation as they have a high purchasing power but lower prices and more choice. They have high demanding power, especially in rich nations, and always request the newest and best developed product. Therefore, knowledge creation can be seen as a major strategic ability for gaining competitive advantage for a company or a nation (Roth, 2003). Due to the fact that Southeast Asia is now continually increasing its investment in R&D, some Asian countries like South Korea will soon transfer from a knowledge development to a knowledge creating country.

Germany puts high emphasis on knowledge creation and innovation. The pharmaceutical industry is the most invested industry in terms of R&D. The successful economical situation can partly be lead back to Germanys' investment in knowledge and, apart from the pharmaceutical, to other successful industries like electrical engineering, chemical industry and motor vehicle industry.

6. Bibliography

Books

Grossman G., M. and Helpman, E. (1991) *Innovation and Growth in the Global Economy.* MIT Press. UK

Krugman, P., R. and Obstfeld, M. (1992) *International Economics – Theory & Policy.* 3rd Ed. HarperCollins College Publishers, NY

Lawler, K. and Seddighi, H. (2001) *International Economics, Theories, Themes and Debates.* Financial Times Prentice Hall.UK

Nonaka, I. and Takeushi, I. (1995) *The knowledge-creating company.* Oxford University Press: New York.

Salvatore, D. (2004) *International Economics,* 8th Ed. John Wiley & Sons. USA

Van Marrewijk, C. (2002) *International Trade & The World Economy.* Oxford University Press. New York

Journals

Bolisani, E. and Scarso, E. (1996) *International Manufacturing Strategies: Experiences from the clothing industry.* International Journal of Operations & Production Management, Vol. 16 No. 11, 1996, pp. 71-84

Cantwell, J. (1995) *The globalisation of technology: what remains of the product cycle model?* Cambridge Journal of Economics. No. 19. pp. 155 -174.

Roth, J. (2003) Enabling *Knowledge Creation: Learning from an R&D organization.* Journal of Knowledge Management. Vol. 7. NO.1, pp. 32 – 48

The Economist (2006) The World in 2006. Countries – The World in figures. The Economist Newspaper Limited. p.106

World-wide R&D (2006) *Innovations - Widening recognition of R&D importance.* Strategic Direction. Vol.22 No.3 pp. 30 - 32

Others

Ambrecht, R. (2006) AAAS Report XXX Research and Development FY 2006. R&D and Innovation in Industry

Federal Ministry of Education and Research (2005) *Research and Innovation in Germany 2005 - Update of the statistical part of the Federal Government's Report on*

Research 2004 .Bundesministerium für Bildung und Forschung / Federal Ministry of Education and Research (BMBF)

Publications and Website Division. Berlin

Pascha, W. (2002) Economic *Realations Between Germany and Japan – An Analysis of Recent Data*. Duisburger Arbeitspapiere zur Ostasienwirtschaft. No.

VFA – Verband Forscher Arzneimittelhersteller ev. (2005) German Association of Research-based Pharmaceutical Companies (VFA) - The pharmaceutical Industry in Germany

Kastelli, J. (2006) *Organisational Knowledge Creation in the Context of R&D cooperation. The role of absorptive capacity*. Paper prepared for the DRUID Winter Conference 2006. National Technical University of Athens

Internet Sources

Tubbs, M. (July, 2005) *Analysis of Global and UK R&D Investments*. www.innovation.gov.uk. Access: 25 June 2006

Invest in Germany (2004) *Germany's Pharmaceutical Industry*. www.invest-in-germany.de. Access: 30 June 2006

UNESCO (2006)

- *Unesco Science Report 2005. Asia overtakes Europe in R&D expenditure -* Updated; 20 February 2006: www.uis.unesco.org. Access: 27 June 2006
- UIS Bulletin on Science and Technology Statistics. (April 2004) *A Decade of Investment in Research and Development (R&D): 1990-2000*. No 1: www.uis.unesco.org. Access: 27 June 2006
-

United Nations (2006)

- Definition of R&D: www.unstats.un.org. Access: 26 June 2006
- World Investment Report 2005. United Nations Conference on Trade and Development: www.unctad.org. Access: 28 June 2006

OECD (2006)

- Factbook 2006 : www.titania.sourceoecd.org. Access: 26 June 2006

VFA - Verband Forschender Arzneimittelhersteller (2006)

- The Pharmaceutical Industry and Innovation: www.vfa.de. Access: 29 June 2006

APPENDIX

Appendix 1:

Gross domestic expenditure on R&D of OECD countries

Gross domestic expenditure on R&D
As a percentage of GDP

	1991	1992	1993	1994	1995	1996	1997	1998	1999	2000	2001	2002	2003	2004
Australia	..	1.52	..	1.50	..	1.67	..	1.51	..	1.56	..	1.69	..	..
Austria	1.44	1.42	1.44	1.51	1.54	1.59	1.69	1.77	1.88	1.91	2.03	2.12	2.19	2.26
Belgium	1.62	..	1.70	1.69	1.72	1.80	1.87	1.90	1.96	2.00	2.11	1.96	1.89	..
Canada	1.60	1.64	1.70	1.76	1.72	1.68	1.68	1.79	1.82	1.93	2.08	1.97	1.95	1.93
Czech Republic	1.90	1.62	1.14	1.03	0.95	0.98	1.09	1.17	1.16	1.23	1.22	1.22	1.26	1.28
Denmark	1.61	1.64	1.72	..	1.82	1.84	1.92	2.04	2.18	..	2.39	2.53	2.62	..
Finland	2.02	2.11	2.14	2.26	2.26	2.52	2.69	2.86	3.21	3.38	3.38	3.43	3.48	..
France	2.33	2.33	2.37	2.32	2.29	2.27	2.19	2.14	2.16	2.15	2.20	2.23	2.18	2.16
Germany	2.47	2.35	2.28	2.18	2.19	2.19	2.24	2.27	2.40	2.45	2.46	2.49	2.52	2.49
Greece	0.36	..	0.47	..	0.49	..	0.51	..	0.67	..	0.65	..	0.62	..
Hungary	1.06	1.04	0.97	0.88	0.73	0.65	0.72	0.68	0.69	0.80	0.95	1.02	0.95	0.88
Iceland	1.18	1.36	1.37	1.41	1.58	..	1.89	2.08	2.39	2.76	3.08	3.14	2.97	..
Ireland	0.93	1.04	1.17	1.27	1.28	1.32	1.29	1.25	1.19	1.14	1.11	1.12	1.19	1.21
Italy	1.23	1.18	1.13	1.05	1.00	1.01	1.05	1.07	1.04	1.07	1.11	1.16	..	..
Japan	2.76	2.71	2.63	2.58	2.69	2.78	2.84	2.95	2.96	2.99	3.07	3.12	3.15	..
Korea	1.84	1.94	2.12	2.32	2.37	2.42	2.48	2.34	2.25	2.39	2.59	2.53	2.63	..
Luxembourg	..	..	..	..	..	..	..	..	..	1.71	..	..	1.78	..
Mexico	..	..	0.22	0.29	0.31	0.31	0.34	0.38	0.43	0.37	0.39	..	..	..
Netherlands	1.97	1.90	1.93	1.97	1.99	2.01	2.04	1.94	2.02	1.90	1.88	1.80	1.84	..
New Zealand	0.98	1.00	1.01	..	0.96	..	1.10	..	1.01	..	1.15	..	1.16	..
Norway	1.64	..	1.72	..	1.70	..	1.64	..	1.65	..	1.60	1.67	1.75	..
Poland	0.76	0.78	0.78	0.71	0.65	0.67	0.67	0.68	0.70	0.66	0.64	0.58	0.56	..
Portugal	0.57	0.61	0.61	0.59	0.57	0.60	0.62	0.69	0.75	0.80	0.85	0.80	0.78	..
Slovak Republic	2.13	1.78	1.38	0.90	0.93	0.92	1.09	0.79	0.66	0.65	0.64	0.58	0.58	0.53
Spain	0.81	0.85	0.85	0.79	0.79	0.80	0.79	0.87	0.86	0.91	0.92	0.99	1.05	..
Sweden	2.72	..	3.17	..	3.35	..	3.54	..	3.65	..	4.29	..	3.98	..
Switzerland	..	2.59	..	..	..	2.67	..	..	..	2.57	..	..	..	..
Turkey	0.53	0.49	0.44	0.36	0.38	0.45	0.49	0.50	0.63	0.64	0.72	0.66	..	..
United Kingdom	2.07	2.03	2.06	2.01	1.95	1.88	1.81	1.80	1.87	1.86	1.87	1.89	1.88	..
United States	2.71	2.64	2.52	2.42	2.51	2.55	2.58	2.62	2.66	2.74	2.76	2.65	2.68	2.68
EU15	1.87	1.85	1.84	1.80	1.78	1.78	1.78	1.79	1.84	1.87	1.90	1.91	1.91	..
OECD total	2.20	2.16	2.11	2.06	2.08	2.10	2.13	2.15	2.19	2.23	2.28	2.24	2.26	..
Brazil	..	..	..	..	..	..	..	..	..	0.99	1.02	0.98	0.95	0.93
China	0.74	0.74	0.72	0.65	0.60	0.60	0.68	0.70	0.83	1.00	1.07	1.22	1.31	1.44
India	..	..	..	..	..	..	..	0.61	0.67	0.72	0.78	..	..	..
Russian Federation	1.43	0.74	0.77	0.84	0.85	0.97	1.04	0.95	1.00	1.05	1.18	1.25	1.29	1.17
South Africa	0.84	..	0.61	..	..	..	0.60	..	..	..	0.73	..	..	..

StatLink: http://dx.doi.org/10.1787/315080082477

Source: OECD Factbook, 2006

Appendix 2:

Gross domestic expenditure on R&D in Germany

I.1 Gross domestic expenditure on R&D (GERD) in Germany absolute and as share of gross domestic product (GDP)

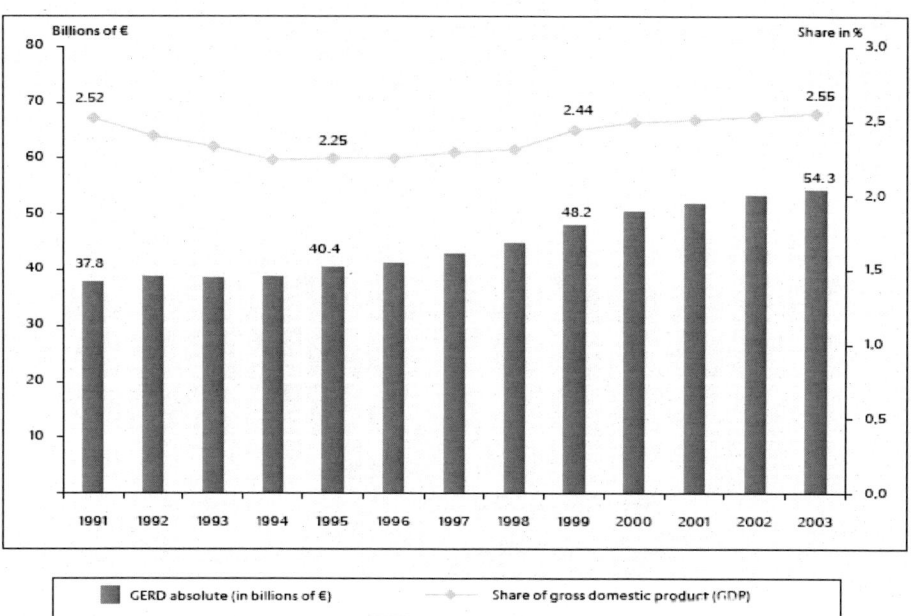

Source: Federal Ministry of Education and Research, 2005

Appendix 3:

Expenditure on education, science, research and development by the Federal Ministry of Education and Research

I.2 Expenditure on education, science, research and development by the Federal Ministry of Education and Research (BMBF) 1991 - 2005

- Billions of € -

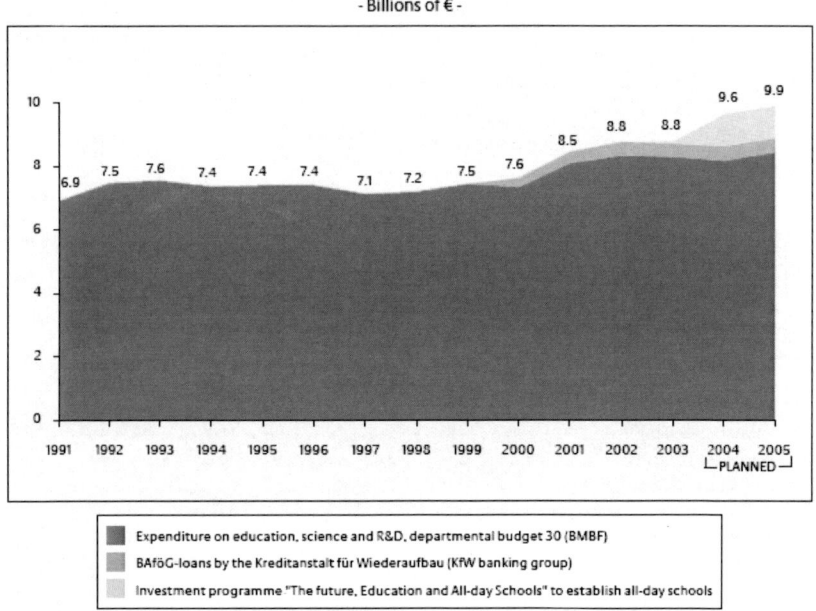

Source: Federal Ministry of Education and Research, 2005

Appendix 4:

R&D Intensity in Germany in 2002

R&D Intensity

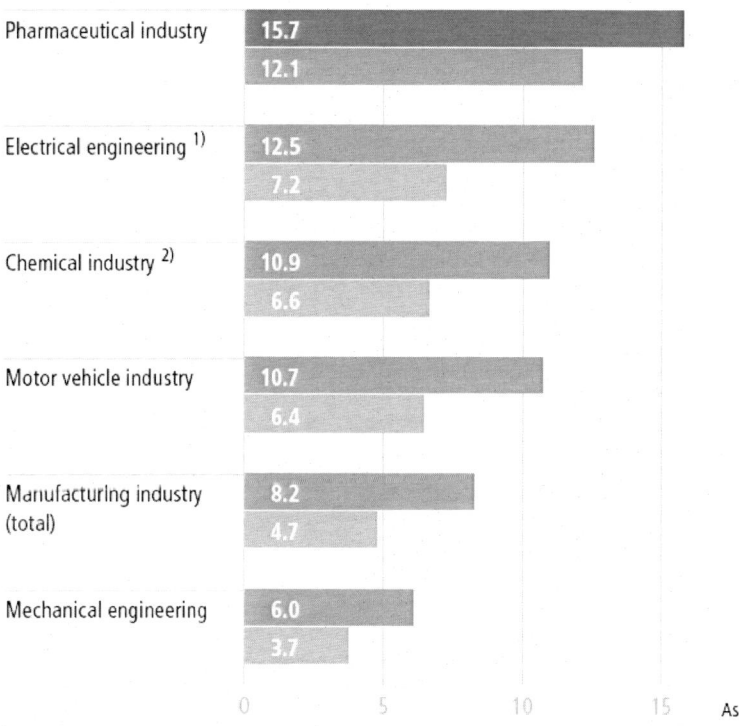

R&D employees in percent of total employees

R&D expenditures in percent of sales

Pharmaceutical industry	15.7 / 12.1
Electrical engineering [1]	12.5 / 7.2
Chemical industry [2]	10.9 / 6.6
Motor vehicle industry	10.7 / 6.4
Manufacturing industry (total)	8.2 / 4.7
Mechanical engineering	6.0 / 3.7

As of: 2001

Source: VFA, 2005

Appendix 5:

Pharmaceutical Industry in Germany – Facts and Figures 2004

1. Pharmaceutical Industry

Sales volume	Total	23.70	EUR billion
	includes foreign sales worth	13.10	EUR billion
	Export rate	55	percent
Capital spending	Research-based pharma. comp. (VFA)	1.36	EUR billion
Employees	Pharmaceutical industry in total	114,200	
	Research-based pharma. comp. (VFA)	84,600	
Price trend	SHI pharmaceuticals	−3	percent
1988 to 2004	Cost of living	+ 42	percent
Price structure	Manufacturer's share in retail price	55	percent

2. Research and Development (R&D)

New molecular entities	Market launch 2004	35	
R&D expenditures	Research-based pharma. comp. (VFA)	3.90	EUR billion
R&D employees	Research-based pharma. comp. (VFA)	14,500	
Research and development	Average cost	800	US-$ million
of a new medicine	Average R&D period	12	years
Genetically manufactured	Germany's share in the total number		
substances	of patent applications	11	percent

3. Pharmaceuticals in the Health Care System

Pharmaceutical	Share in gross domestic product 2004	1.7	percent
expenditures	Share in health care spending 2004	15.7	percent
	Share in health care spending 1992	15.9	percent
SHI	Total expenditures	139.9	EUR billion
	includes pharma. expenditures worth	21.8	EUR billion
	in percent of total expenditures	15.6	percent
SHI pharmaceutical prices	Change over previous year	− 2.4	percent

4. German Pharmaceutical Market

Number of pharmaceuticals	90% of all prescriptions are issued for	2,200	pharmaceuticals
Per-capita consumption	Packages	17.7	
Pharmacy market	Sales at manufacturers' prices	18.0	EUR billion
	Prescription drugs	14.8	EUR billion
	Prescribed OTC drugs	0.8	EUR billion
	Self-medication	2.4	EUR billion
Innovative pharmaceuticals	Sales share of new molecular entities during the past 5 years	7.5	percent
Generics	Sales share in the SHI market eligible for generic drugs	68	percent
Reference prices	Share of prescriptions in the SHI market	62	percent
Parallel imports	Sales share in the pharmacy market	5	percent

5. The International Pharmaceutical Market

Worldwide sales	Total	550	Mrd. US-$
	Share of German sales 2004	4	Prozent
	Share of German sales 1997	5	Prozent
Per-capita sales 2003	Germany	250	US-$
In comparison:	USA	552	US-$
	Japan	345	US-$
	France	298	US-$
	United Kingdom	205	US-$

Source: VFA, 2005